The Mindful Kitchen:
Nourishing Recipes and Practices for a Healthier Relationship with Food

By

Tommy Blair

Table of Contents

Introduction

Welcome to **"The Mindful Kitchen: Nourishing Recipes and Practices for a Healthier Relationship with Food"**.

In today's fast-paced world, it's easy to get caught up in the rush of everyday life and forget to slow down and appreciate the small things - including our food. Mindful eating is a practice that can help us reconnect with our bodies and the food we consume, leading to a healthier relationship with food and ourselves.

In this book, you'll learn about the benefits of mindful eating and how to incorporate it into your daily life. You'll discover how to set up your kitchen for mindful eating, reduce food waste, and create a calming environment. You'll also find practical exercises and meditations to help you become more mindful of your eating habits and cultivate a deeper connection with your body.

Additionally, this book provides a collection of nourishing and delicious recipes for every meal, from breakfast to dessert, that can be enjoyed mindfully. You'll also find tips for mindful eating on the go and how to handle emotional eating triggers during special occasions.

By the end of this book, you'll have the tools and knowledge necessary to make mindful eating a part of your daily routine. Let's begin the journey towards a healthier relationship with food and ourselves.

What is mindful eating?

Mindful eating is the practice of paying attention to the experience of eating, with all your senses, and without judgment. It involves being fully present and engaged with the food you're eating, as well as with the process of eating itself.

This means taking the time to savor each bite, noticing the flavors, textures, and aromas of your food, and paying attention to how your body responds to what you're eating. Mindful eating also involves becoming more aware of your hunger and fullness cues and eating in a way that honors those cues.

By practicing mindful eating, you can develop a deeper connection with your body, improve your relationship with food, and make more conscious and nourishing food choices. Mindful eating can also help you become more aware of emotional and environmental triggers that affect your eating habits, and empower you to make healthier choices.

Why is it important?

Mindful eating is important for several reasons.

Here are a few key ones:

- **Promotes a healthier relationship with food**

Mindful eating helps you develop a more positive and balanced relationship with food. By paying attention to your body's cues and eating in a way that honors them, you can learn to trust your body and make more nourishing food choices.

- **Helps prevent overeating**

When you eat mindfully, you become more aware of your body's hunger and fullness signals. This can help you avoid overeating or eating past the point of fullness.

- **Reduces stress and improves mental health**

Mindful eating can help reduce stress and improve your overall mental health. By being fully present and engaged with your food, you can cultivate a sense of calm and relaxation during meal times.

- **Enhances digestion**

When you eat mindfully, you give your body the time and space it needs to properly digest your food. This can lead to improved digestion and absorption of nutrients.

- **Supports weight management**

Mindful eating can support healthy weight management by helping you make more conscious and nourishing food choices, and by preventing overeating.

Overall, mindful eating is a powerful tool for improving your relationship with food, enhancing your physical and mental well-being, and promoting a healthier, more balanced lifestyle.

How can it benefit you?

Practicing mindful eating can benefit you in a number of ways.

Below are some of the main benefits:

- **Improves digestion**

By taking the time to fully chew and savor your food, you can help your body digest your meals more efficiently, leading to better nutrient absorption and a reduced risk of digestive issues like bloating and constipation.

- **Supports weight management**

Mindful eating can help you become more aware of your hunger and fullness cues, which can help you make more conscious and nourishing food choices, and prevent overeating.

- **Promotes a healthier relationship with food**

Mindful eating can help you develop a more positive and balanced relationship with food. By becoming more aware of the flavors, textures, and aromas of your meals, you can learn to appreciate food as a source of nourishment and pleasure, rather than as a source of guilt or shame.

- **Reduces stress and improves mental health**

Mindful eating can help reduce stress and promote relaxation. By being fully present and engaged with your food, you can cultivate a sense of calm during meal times.

- **Increases mindful awareness**

Practicing mindful eating can help you become more mindful and present in other areas of your life as well. By training your mind to focus on the present moment, you can become more attuned to your thoughts, feelings, and surroundings.

Overall, mindful eating is a powerful tool for improving your physical and mental well-being and promoting a healthier, more balanced lifestyle.

Chapter 1

The Mindful Kitchen

"The Mindful Kitchen" refers to the concept of applying mindfulness to the act of cooking and preparing food. It involves bringing a sense of awareness, presence, and intention to the kitchen, creating a space where cooking becomes a mindful and meditative practice.

In the mindful kitchen, every step of the cooking process is approached with attention and care. From selecting ingredients mindfully to chopping vegetables with focus and precision, to appreciating the smells and textures that arise during cooking, each action is performed with a sense of mindfulness and presence.

The mindful kitchen is not just about the end result—the delicious and nourishing meals that are prepared—but also about the process itself. It's about cultivating a deeper connection with the food we eat, honoring the ingredients, and being fully engaged in the act of nourishing ourselves and others.

By practicing mindfulness in the kitchen, we can transform cooking from a mundane chore into a meaningful and enjoyable experience. The mindful kitchen becomes a place of creativity, self-expression, and self-care, where the act of preparing food becomes a source of joy, satisfaction, and connection with ourselves and the world around us.

How to set up your kitchen for mindful eating

Setting up your kitchen for mindful eating involves creating an environment that supports and encourages mindful food choices and eating habits.

Here are some tips to help you set up your kitchen for mindful eating:

- **Clear and organized space**

Start by decluttering your kitchen and creating a clean, organized space. A clutter-free environment can promote a sense of calm and make it easier to focus on the present moment while preparing and enjoying your meals.

- **Mindful food storage**

Arrange your pantry, refrigerator, and cabinets in a way that promotes mindful food choices. Keep healthier options, such as fresh fruits, vegetables, whole grains, and nuts, at eye level and within easy reach. Place less nutritious or indulgent foods in less accessible areas.

- **Mindful kitchen tools**

Invest in kitchen tools that support your mindful eating goals. For example, a good set of knives, cutting boards, and quality cookware can make food preparation more enjoyable and precise. Consider tools that encourage slow cooking methods, such as a slow cooker or a steamer, to cultivate a mindful approach to meal preparation.

- **Minimal distractions**

Minimize distractions in your kitchen to promote a more focused and present cooking and eating experience. Keep electronic devices, such as phones and tablets, out of the kitchen or set them to silent mode. Avoid multitasking while eating, such as watching TV or working on your computer, and instead, create a dedicated space for mindful meals.

- **Mindful dining area**

Set up a designated space for mindful eating. This can be a cozy corner of your kitchen or a separate dining area. Use mindful eating cues such as a simple table setting, beautiful placemats, and perhaps a centerpiece like fresh flowers or a candle to create a visually appealing and inviting space for your meals.

- **Mindful reminders**

Place visual reminders of mindful eating in your kitchen. You can hang inspirational quotes, mindfulness sayings, or even a vision board that represents your health and wellness goals. These reminders can serve as prompts to stay present and make conscious choices while preparing and enjoying your meals.

Remember, setting up your kitchen for mindful eating is about creating an environment that supports your intentions and encourages mindful food choices. Tailor your kitchen space to reflect your personal preferences and cultivate a sense of mindfulness and nourishment as you cook and eat.

Tips for mindful grocery shopping

Mindful grocery shopping involves approaching your shopping experience with awareness and intention and making conscious choices that align with your health and well-being.

Here are some tips to help you practice mindful grocery shopping:

- **Make a shopping list**

Before heading to the grocery store, create a shopping list based on your meal plan and desired healthy food choices. This helps you stay focused and prevents impulsive purchases.

- **Shop with a clear mind**

Avoid grocery shopping when you're hungry, tired, or stressed. These states of mind can lead to impulsive and unhealthy food choices. Take a few moments to calm your mind before heading to the store.

- **Choose whole, unprocessed foods**

Focus on selecting whole, unprocessed foods such as fruits, vegetables, whole grains, lean proteins, and nuts. These foods tend to be more nutrient-dense and support a healthy diet.

- **Read labels mindfully**

When selecting packaged foods, read the labels mindfully. Look for ingredients that align with your health goals and be aware of added sugars, unhealthy fats, and artificial additives. Understanding what you're putting into your body can help you make informed choices.

- **Shop the perimeter**

The perimeter of the grocery store often houses fresh produce, meats, and dairy products. Spend more time in these sections as they typically contain the least processed and most nutritious options. Minimize time in the center aisles where processed foods are often found.

- **Take your time and savor the experience**

Slow down while shopping. Take time to look at the variety of fruits, vegetables, and other foods available. Appreciate the colors, textures, and aromas. Engage your senses and savor the experience of selecting nourishing foods.

• Practice mindful budgeting

Consider your budget as part of mindful shopping. Opt for cost-effective healthy options and prioritize your spending on foods that provide maximum nutritional value. You can also explore local farmers' markets or bulk food sections for affordable and fresh options.

• Be mindful of portion sizes

When purchasing items, be mindful of portion sizes. Consider your actual needs and avoid buying excessive quantities that may lead to food waste or overconsumption.

• Engage with the environment

Pay attention to the environmental impact of your choices. Opt for products with minimal packaging or choose reusable options. Support local and sustainable food sources when possible.

Remember, mindful grocery shopping is about cultivating awareness and making conscious choices that align with your health and well-being. By approaching your shopping experience with mindfulness, you can create a more nourishing and satisfying relationship with the food you bring into your home.

Reducing food waste through mindfulness

Reducing food waste is not only beneficial for the environment but also aligns with mindful eating principles. Mindfulness can help us become more aware of our food consumption habits and make conscious choices to minimize waste.

Here are some tips for reducing food waste through mindfulness:

- **Plan meals and create a shopping list**

Plan your meals for the week ahead and create a shopping list based on those plans. This helps you buy only what you need and reduces the chances of purchasing excess food that may go to waste.

- **Buy and use perishables wisely**

Be mindful of perishable items like fruits, vegetables, and dairy products. Consider their shelf life and plan to use them before they spoil. Opt for smaller quantities if you know you won't consume them in time.

- **Practice proper food storage**

Take care to store food properly to maintain freshness and extend its shelf life. Follow recommended storage guidelines for different types of produce, and use airtight containers or wraps to keep food fresh.

- **Practice the first-in, first-out approach**

Organize your fridge and pantry to ensure older items are used before newer ones. This reduces the likelihood of food items expiring or being forgotten.

- **Embrace leftovers creatively**

Leftovers can be transformed into delicious meals with a little creativity. Instead of discarding them, repurpose leftovers into new dishes or use them for lunches the next day.

- **Practice mindful portion control**

Serve yourself reasonable portions to avoid excess food ending up in the trash. You can always go back for more food if you are still hungry.

- **Get creative with scraps**

Instead of discarding vegetable scraps like peels or stems, consider using them to make homemade stocks, soups, or vegetable broth. Fruit peels can be used for making infused water or used as compost.

- **Freeze and preserve**

If you have excess fruits, vegetables, or meals that you won't be able to consume in time, consider freezing them for later use. Properly labeled and stored frozen foods can extend their shelf life significantly.

- **Practice mindful consumption**

Be conscious of your eating habits and avoid mindless snacking or buying more food than necessary. Mindful eating encourages us to be present, savor each bite, and eat until we're satisfied but not excessively full.

By incorporating these mindful practices into your daily routine, you can significantly reduce food waste and contribute to a more sustainable and mindful approach to eating.

Creating a calming kitchen environment

Creating a calming kitchen environment can enhance your overall cooking and dining experience, making it a more enjoyable and mindful space.

Here are some tips to create a calming kitchen environment:

- **Declutter and organize**

Start by decluttering your kitchen and keeping countertops clear of unnecessary items. Remove any visual distractions that can create a sense of chaos or overwhelm. Organize your kitchen tools, utensils, and ingredients in a way that is neat and easily accessible.

- **Soft lighting**

Opt for soft, warm lighting in your kitchen to create a cozy and calming atmosphere. Use dimmable lights or add ambient lighting options such as pendant lights, under-cabinet lighting, or even candles to create a soothing ambiance.

- **Natural elements**

Incorporate natural elements into your kitchen space to bring a sense of calm and grounding. Place a vase of fresh flowers, a small potted plant, or a bowl of fresh fruits on the countertop. Consider adding natural materials like wooden cutting boards, bamboo utensils, or stone countertops.

- **Aromatherapy**

Utilize the power of scents to create a calming environment. Use essential oils or natural scented candles with relaxing fragrances such as lavender, chamomile, or citrus. The pleasant aromas can help reduce stress and create a soothing atmosphere in your kitchen.

- **Music or soothing sounds**

Play soft, calming music or nature sounds while cooking or enjoying meals. Gentle instrumental music or sounds of nature can create a serene and peaceful ambiance in your kitchen.

- **Mindful decor**

Select kitchen decor that promotes a sense of mindfulness and tranquility. Hang inspirational or calming artwork on the walls, and display meaningful quotes or phrases related to food, health, or mindfulness. These visual reminders can contribute to a serene and mindful atmosphere.

- **Cleanliness and simplicity**

Keep your kitchen clean and organized on a regular basis. A clean and clutter-free space promotes a sense of calm and relaxation. Simplify your kitchen tools and gadgets, keeping only the essentials within reach.

- **Mindful rituals**

Incorporate mindful rituals into your kitchen routine. Take a moment to pause and appreciate the ingredients before cooking. Practice gratitude for the nourishing food you are preparing. Engage in mindful breathing or a short meditation while waiting for the water to boil or food to cook.

Remember, creating a calming kitchen environment is about designing a space that supports your mindful eating and cooking practices. Customizing your kitchen to be a peaceful and harmonious space can enhance your overall well-being and make your time in the kitchen a more enjoyable and mindful experience.

Chapter 2

Mindful Eating Practices

Mindful eating practices involve bringing awareness, presence, and intention to the act of eating. By incorporating these practices into your meals, you can cultivate a deeper connection with your food, your body, and the overall eating experience.

Here are some mindful eating practices to consider:

- **Slow down**

Eat at a slower pace and savor each bite. Take the time to chew your food thoroughly and appreciate the flavors, textures, and aromas. This allows you to fully experience and enjoy your meals.

- **Engage your senses**

Pay attention to the sensory aspects of your food. Notice the colors, smells, and sounds. Take delight in the taste and texture of each bite. Engaging your senses helps to anchor you in the present moment.

- **Eat without distractions**

Minimize distractions during meal times. Avoid eating in front of screens, such as the TV, computer, or phone. Instead, create a dedicated space for mindful eating, free from distractions, where you can fully focus on your food.

- **Tune into hunger and fullness cues**

Before eating, check in with your body to assess your level of hunger. Similarly, during your meal, pay attention to your body's signals of fullness. Eat till you're satisfied but not overstuffed.

- **Non-judgmental awareness**

Cultivate non-judgmental awareness of your thoughts, feelings, and reactions while eating. Notice any judgments or negative thoughts that arise and let them go. Approach your food with a sense of curiosity and acceptance.

- **Gratitude and appreciation**

Express gratitude for the food you are about to eat. Reflect on the efforts that went into growing, preparing, and bringing the food to your plate. Develop a sense of appreciation for the nourishment it provides.

- **Mindful portioning**

Serve yourself mindful portions that align with your hunger and nutritional needs. Consider the balance of different food groups and aim for a variety of colors and nutrients on your plate.

- **Cultivate mindful cooking**

Extend mindfulness to the cooking process itself. Engage in the preparation of your meals with focus, intention, and gratitude. Pay attention to the ingredients, the smells, and the actions involved in cooking.

- **Reflect on food choices**

Consider the origins and impacts of your food choices. Connect with the sources of your food, such as local farmers or sustainable practices. Make choices that align with your values and promote your well-being.

- **Practice self-compassion**

Approach mindful eating with self-compassion and kindness. Be gentle with yourself if you have challenging moments or slip-ups. Remember that mindful eating is a practice, and it's about progress, not perfection.

By incorporating these mindful eating practices into your daily life, you can develop a healthier and more balanced relationship with food, savor the pleasure of eating, and cultivate a greater sense of well-being.

Mindful eating exercises and meditations

Practicing mindful eating exercises and meditations can deepen your awareness and connection with the eating experience.

Here are a few exercises and meditations you can try:

Mindful Eating Meditation:

- Find a quiet and comfortable space to sit down with your meal.
- Take a few deep breaths to ground yourself and bring your attention to the present moment.
- Begin by observing the appearance of your food, noticing the colors, shapes, and textures.
- Take a moment to appreciate the aroma of the food, inhaling deeply and savoring the scents.
- Slowly take your first bite, paying attention to the sensations in your mouth as you chew.

- Notice the taste, the texture, and the temperature of the food.
- Chew slowly and thoroughly, taking your time with each bite.
- As you continue to eat, stay present with each sensation, observing any thoughts or emotions that arise.
- Cultivate a sense of gratitude for the nourishment and pleasure that the food brings.
- Take breaks between bites, pausing to check in with your body's hunger and fullness cues.
- Continue eating mindfully until you feel satisfied and content.

Raisin Exercise:

- Take a single raisin or any small piece of food and hold it in your hand.
- Observe the raisin as if you've never seen one before. Notice its color, texture, and shape.
- Bring the raisin close to your nose and inhale its aroma. Take note of any scents or associations that arise.

- Place the raisin in your mouth without chewing it right away. Explore its texture, weight, and temperature as it rests on your tongue.
- Slowly begin to chew the raisin, paying attention to the movement of your jaw and the release of flavors.
- Notice the changing texture as you continue to chew. Be fully present with the sensations in your mouth.
- Swallow the raisin and feel it moving down your throat.
- Take a moment to reflect on the experience, noticing any thoughts or emotions that emerged during the exercise.

Mindful Savoring:

- Select a small piece of your favorite food or a treat that you enjoy.
- Take a moment to observe the food, noticing its appearance and any anticipation or excitement that arises.
- Take a small bite and hold it in your mouth without chewing right away.

- Close your eyes if it helps you to focus more on the flavors and sensations.
- Allow the flavors to gradually unfold as you slowly chew the food.
- Notice the different tastes, textures, and sensations that emerge with each bite.
- Pay attention to any shifts or changes in the flavors as you continue to savor the food.
- Take your time to fully experience and enjoy the taste, savoring the moment.
- When ready, swallow the food and observe any aftertastes or lingering sensations.
- Take a moment to appreciate the experience and express gratitude for the pleasure of savoring the food.

These exercises and meditations can help cultivate a deeper sense of presence, awareness, and appreciation for the food you consume. Practice them regularly to enhance your mindful eating journey and develop a more conscious and enjoyable relationship with your meals.

Eating with all your senses

Eating with all your senses is a practice of engaging and fully experiencing the sensory aspects of food. By tuning in to your senses while eating, you can enhance your appreciation for the flavors, textures, aromas, and visual appeal of your meals.

Here's how you can eat with all your senses:

Sight:

- Take a moment to visually appreciate your food before you start eating.
- Notice the colors, shapes, and arrangement of the food on your plate.
- Observe any vibrant or contrasting colors present.
- Pay attention to the visual appeal of the presentation.

Smell:

- Bring the food close to your nose and take a deep breath.

- Notice the aromas and scents that arise.
- Take a moment to identify and appreciate the various smells.
- Allow the aromas to awaken your anticipation and appetite.

Touch:

- Feel the texture of the food with your fingertips or hands.
- Notice the temperature, whether it's warm, cold, or at room temperature.
- Pay attention to the surface, whether it's smooth, rough, or crispy.
- Experience the tactile sensations as you handle the food and bring it to your mouth.

Sound:

- Listen to the sounds associated with your food.
- Notice any sizzling, crackling, or crunching sounds.

- Pay attention to the sounds you make while chewing and the texture-related noises.
- Be present with the auditory experience of your meal.

Taste:

- Savor the flavors in your mouth by taking small bites.
- Pay attention to the different tastes, such as sweet, salty, sour, bitter, and umami.
- Notice the complexity and nuances of the flavors.
- Explore how the taste evolves as you continue to chew and swallow.

Mindful chewing:

- Chew slowly and thoroughly, allowing the food to mix with saliva.
- Notice the sensation of chewing, the movement of your jaw, and the texture of the food.

- Be fully present with the act of chewing and the changes that occur as the food breaks down.
- Take your time to savor each bite before swallowing.

By engaging all your senses while eating, you can cultivate a deeper connection with your food and the present moment. It enhances the pleasure and satisfaction of the eating experience, allowing you to fully appreciate the sensory aspects of the food you consume. Incorporate this practice into your meals to make them more enjoyable, mindful, and satisfying.

How to identify and honor your hunger and fullness cues

Identifying and honoring your hunger and fullness cues is an important aspect of mindful eating. Tuning in to your body's signals can help you make more conscious choices about when to eat, how much to eat, and when to stop.

Here are some tips to help you identify and honor your hunger and fullness cues:

- **Check-in with yourself**

Throughout the day, take a moment to pause and check in with your body. Ask yourself how hungry or full you feel on a scale from 1 to 10, where 1 is extremely hungry and 10 is overly full.

- **Notice physical sensations**

Pay attention to the physical sensations in your body that indicate hunger. This could include stomach growling, a hollow feeling in your stomach, low energy, lightheadedness, or difficulty concentrating.

- **Distinguish between physical and emotional cues**

Learn to differentiate between physical hunger and emotional hunger. Physical hunger arises gradually and is accompanied by physical sensations, while emotional hunger tends to come on suddenly and is often triggered by specific emotions or situations.

- **Eat when you feel moderately hungry**

Aim to eat when you feel moderately hungry (around a 3 or 4 on the hunger scale). Waiting until you are ravenous can lead to overeating, while eating when you're only slightly hungry may not fully satisfy your body's needs.

- **Eat mindfully**

When you do eat, engage in mindful eating practices as mentioned earlier. Slow down, savor each bite, and pay attention to your body's signals as you eat. This allows you to notice when you're starting to feel satisfied.

- **Pause during meals**

Take breaks during your meal to check in with your body's fullness cues. Put your utensils down, take a deep breath, and assess how satisfied you feel.

Notice any changes in physical sensations, such as feeling less hungry or more comfortable.

• Stop before feeling overly full

Aim to stop eating when you feel comfortably satisfied, around a 6 or 7 on the fullness scale. Avoid the temptation to clean your plate or continue eating out of habit. Trust your body's signals that indicate you've had enough.

• Practice portion control

Be mindful of portion sizes to prevent overeating. Start with smaller portions and listen to your body's cues before going for seconds. You can always have more if you're still hungry, but honoring your fullness is equally important.

• Be patient and forgiving

It takes time and practice to become attuned to your hunger and fullness cues. Be patient with yourself and understand that it's normal to have occasional slips or challenges. Approach this process with self-compassion and a non-judgmental attitude.

By developing awareness of your body's hunger and fullness cues and honoring them, you can establish a healthier relationship with food and support your overall well-being. Listening to your body's wisdom and nourishing it accordingly is an essential aspect of mindful eating.

Mindful portion control

Mindful portion control involves being aware of the amount of food you consume and making conscious choices about serving sizes. It allows you to find a balance between nourishing your body and enjoying your meals.

Below are some tips for practicing mindful portion control:

- **Use visual cues**

Familiarize yourself with visual references for portion sizes. For example, a serving of protein (such as meat or fish) should be about the size of a deck of cards, a serving of pasta or grains can fit in a cupped hand, and a serving of vegetables is roughly the size of your fist. Visualizing these references can help you estimate appropriate portion sizes.

- **Read food labels**

Pay close attention to serving sizes listed on food labels. Compare the serving size to the amount you typically eat, and adjust accordingly. Be mindful of the number of servings per container, as sometimes a package may contain multiple servings.

- **Use smaller plates and bowls**

Opt for smaller plates and bowls to help control portion sizes. When you use a smaller plate, it can create the perception of a fuller plate, which may help you feel satisfied with a smaller amount of food.

- **Serve yourself mindfully**

When serving your meals, start with smaller portions and pay attention to your hunger and fullness cues. You can always go back for seconds if you're still hungry, but this allows you to assess your level of satisfaction before automatically reaching for more.

- **Be mindful of high-calorie foods**

Be particularly mindful of portion sizes when it comes to high-calorie foods, such as desserts, snacks, or foods with added fats and sugars. These items tend to have a higher energy density, meaning they contain more calories in a smaller volume, so portion control is important.

- **Practice mindful eating**

Engage in mindful eating practices as mentioned earlier, such as eating slowly, savoring each bite, and paying attention to your body's fullness cues. This can help you become more aware of when you've had enough, preventing overeating.

● Prioritize vegetables and whole foods

Fill a significant portion of your plate with vegetables and whole foods. These nutrient-dense options are generally lower in calories and higher in fiber, helping you feel more satisfied with reasonable portions.

● Plan and prepare meals in advance

Planning and preparing your meals in advance can help you control portion sizes. By portioning out meals and snacks ahead of time, you're less likely to overindulge or eat mindlessly.

● Listen to your body

Trust your body's signals and listen to its cues for hunger and fullness. Avoid eating out of stress, boredom, or emotions. Tune in to your body's actual needs rather than relying on external cues or portion sizes dictated by others.

Remember, portion control is about finding a balance that works for you and your body's unique needs. It's not about strict deprivation or counting every calorie. By practicing mindful portion control, you can support your health goals while still enjoying a satisfying and nourishing relationship with food.

Chapter 3

Nourishing Recipes for Every Meal

Incorporating nourishing recipes into every meal is a wonderful way to prioritize your health and well-being.

Here are some ideas for nourishing recipes for each meal of the day:

Breakfast:

- **Veggie-packed omelet**

Whip up an omelet with a variety of colorful vegetables like bell peppers, spinach, mushrooms, and tomatoes. To add flavor add some herbs and spices.

- **Overnight oats**

Combine rolled oats, your choice of milk, chia seeds, and a sweetener like honey or maple syrup. Let it sit in the fridge overnight and top it with fresh fruits, nuts, and seeds in the morning.

- **Avocado toast**

Toast a slice of whole-grain bread and top it with mashed avocado, a sprinkle of sea salt, and a squeeze of lemon or lime juice. Optional toppings include sliced tomatoes, micro greens, or a poached egg.

Lunch:

- **Quinoa salad**

Mix cooked quinoa with chopped vegetables, such as cucumbers, cherry tomatoes, bell peppers, and fresh herbs. Dress it with a lemon vinaigrette and add some crumbled feta or grilled chicken for extra protein.

- **Buddha bowl**

Create a nourishing bowl with a base of mixed greens or grains like brown rice or quinoa. Top it with roasted vegetables, legumes (e.g., chickpeas or lentils), avocado slices, and a drizzle of tahini or a homemade dressing.

- **Veggie wrap**

Wrap a whole-grain tortilla with hummus or mashed avocado, and fill it with a variety of sliced vegetables, sprouts, and a source of protein like grilled tofu or sliced turkey.

Dinner:

- **Baked salmon with roasted vegetables**

Season a salmon fillet with herbs, lemon juice, and olive oil, and bake it in the oven. Serve it with a side of roasted vegetables like broccoli, carrots, and Brussels sprouts.

- **Stir-fried tofu and vegetables**

Sauté tofu cubes with a mix of colorful vegetables like bell peppers, snow peas, carrots, and broccoli. Add a flavorful sauce made with soy sauce, ginger, garlic, and a touch of honey or maple syrup.

- **Quinoa-stuffed bell peppers**

Cook a mixture of quinoa, black beans, corn, diced tomatoes, and spices. Stuff the mixture into halved bell peppers, top with cheese if desired, and bake until the peppers are tender.

Snacks:

- **Greek yogurt with berries**

Enjoy a bowl of Greek yogurt topped with fresh berries, a sprinkle of granola, and a drizzle of honey.

- **Vegetable crudité with hummus**

Slice a variety of vegetables like carrots, cucumbers, bell peppers, and cherry tomatoes. Serve with hummus on the side for dipping.

- **Energy balls**

Combine dates, nuts, seeds, and your choice of flavorings like cocoa powder or vanilla extract in a food processor. Roll the mixture into bite-sized balls for a nutritious and portable snack.

These are only a few ideas to get you started. Remember to choose whole, unprocessed ingredients and customize the recipes to suit your taste preferences and dietary needs. Experiment with different flavors and ingredients to make each meal nourishing, delicious, and satisfying.

Mindful breakfast recipes

Starting your day with a mindful breakfast sets a positive tone for the rest of the day.

Here are a few mindful breakfast recipes to inspire you:

Berry and Yogurt Parfait:

- Layer Greek yogurt, mixed berries (such as strawberries, blueberries, and raspberries), and a sprinkle of granola or nuts in a glass or bowl.
- Drizzle with a touch of honey or maple syrup for sweetness.
- Enjoy the creamy, fruity, and crunchy layers mindfully, savoring each bite.

Green Smoothie Bowl:

- In a blender, combine a handful of spinach or kale, a ripe banana, a cup of frozen mixed berries, a spoonful of nut butter, and your choice of milk (such as almond milk or coconut milk).

- Blend until smooth and creamy.
- Pour the smoothie into a bowl and top it with sliced fruits, granola, chia seeds, or shredded coconut.
- Eat it slowly, appreciating the vibrant colors and refreshing flavors.

Avocado and Egg Toast:

- Toast a slice of whole-grain bread.
- Half an avocado, mashed, should be spread on toast.
- Cook an egg (fried, poached, or scrambled) and place it on top of the avocado.
- Sprinkle with salt, pepper, and optional toppings like chopped herbs or red pepper flakes.
- Savor the combination of creamy avocado, protein-rich egg, and crunchy toast mindfully.

Overnight Chia Pudding:

- In a jar, mix 1/4 cup of chia seeds with your choice of milk (such as almond milk or coconut milk), a sweetener like honey or maple syrup, and a dash of vanilla extract.
- Stir well and refrigerate overnight.
- In the morning, give it a good stir and add toppings like fresh fruit, nuts, and a sprinkle of cinnamon.
- Enjoy the smooth, pudding-like texture and the subtle sweetness of the chia seeds.

Whole Grain Pancakes/Waffles:

- Prepare pancakes or waffles using whole grain flour (such as whole wheat or oat flour).
- Serve them with a variety of toppings like fresh fruit, Greek yogurt, a drizzle of pure maple syrup, and a sprinkle of nuts or seeds.
- Take your time to savor each bite, appreciating the fluffy texture and the combination of flavors.

Remember, the key to mindful eating is to engage your senses, eat slowly, and pay attention to the flavors, textures, and nourishment that each bite brings. Customize these recipes based on your preferences and dietary needs, and make sure to choose ingredients that align with your mindful eating goals.

Mindful lunch recipes

Enjoying a mindful lunch can help you recharge and refocus during the day.

Here are a few mindful lunch recipes to inspire you:

Buddha Bowl:

- Start with a base of mixed greens or cooked quinoa.
- Add a variety of colorful vegetables, such as roasted sweet potatoes, sautéed kale, cherry tomatoes, shredded carrots, and sliced cucumbers.
- Top with a source of protein, like grilled chicken, tofu, chickpeas, or cooked lentils.
- Drizzle with a homemade dressing or tahini sauce.
- Take your time to savor each ingredient, appreciating the combination of flavors and textures.

Nourishing Salad Wrap:

- Take a large lettuce leaf or a whole-grain wrap.
- Spread a layer of hummus, Greek yogurt, or mashed avocado on the wrap.
- Fill it with a variety of salad ingredients, such as mixed greens, sliced cucumbers, shredded carrots, cherry tomatoes, and sprouts.
- Add a source of protein like grilled chicken, turkey slices, tofu, or chickpeas.
- Roll it up and enjoy each bite, being mindful of the fresh and crisp flavors.

Quinoa and Vegetable Stir-Fry:

- Cook quinoa according to package instructions.
- In a pan, stir-fry a mix of colorful vegetables like bell peppers, broccoli, snap peas, and mushrooms with a bit of olive oil and your choice of seasoning (such as garlic, ginger, and soy sauce).
- Add the cooked quinoa to the pan and toss to combine.

- Optional: Add a protein source like grilled shrimp, tofu cubes, or edamame.
- Savor the combination of textures and flavors as you enjoy each spoonful mindfully.

Mediterranean Grain Bowl:

- Start with a base of cooked whole grains like bulgur, farro, or brown rice.
- Top it with a mix of Mediterranean-inspired ingredients like cherry tomatoes, cucumbers, kalamata olives, feta cheese, and chopped fresh herbs (such as parsley or mint).
- Drizzle with a lemon-herb dressing or a simple olive oil and lemon juice dressing.
- Optional: Add a protein source like grilled chicken, falafel, or chickpeas.
- Take your time to appreciate the vibrant Mediterranean flavors in each bite.

Soba Noodle Salad:

- Soba noodles should be prepared according to package instructions and rinse with cold water.
- Toss the noodles with a mix of julienned vegetables like carrots, bell peppers, cucumber, and scallions.
- Add a handful of edamame or cooked shrimp for protein.
- Drizzle with a sesame-soy dressing or a ginger-lime dressing.
- Enjoy the refreshing and satisfying combination of flavors and textures mindfully.

Remember to personalize these recipes based on your preferences and dietary needs. Allow yourself the time and space to enjoy your lunch in a calm and relaxed environment, free from distractions. Appreciate the nourishment that each ingredient brings and savor the flavors as you eat mindfully.

Mindful dinner recipes

Enjoying a mindful dinner can help you unwind and end your day on a positive note.

Here are a few mindful dinner recipes to inspire you:

Grilled Salmon with Quinoa and Roasted Vegetables:

- Grill a salmon fillet seasoned with herbs, lemon juice, and olive oil until cooked through.
- Prepare quinoa according to package instructions as a nutritious side dish.
- Roast a variety of vegetables like broccoli, carrots, and Brussels sprouts with a drizzle of olive oil and a sprinkle of sea salt.
- Arrange the grilled salmon, quinoa, and roasted vegetables on a plate and savor the flavors and textures mindfully.

Stuffed Bell Peppers:

- Cut the tops off bell peppers and remove the seeds and membranes.
- In a skillet, sauté diced onions, garlic, and your choice of protein (such as ground turkey or tofu) until cooked through.
- Add cooked quinoa or brown rice, diced tomatoes, and a mix of herbs and spices.
- Fill the bell peppers with the stuffing mixture and bake until the peppers are tender and lightly browned.
- Enjoy the colorful and flavorful stuffed bell peppers, being present with each bite.

Vegetable Stir-Fry with Tofu:

- In a wok or skillet, stir-fry a variety of colorful vegetables like bell peppers, snap peas, carrots, and broccoli with a bit of sesame oil and soy sauce.
- Add cubed tofu and continue cooking until the tofu is heated through.
- Season with your choice of spices, such as ginger, garlic, or chili flakes.

- Serve the vegetable stir-fry over a bed of steamed brown rice or noodles.
- Take your time to appreciate the fresh, vibrant flavors and the nourishment it provides.

Quinoa and Black Bean Salad:

- Allow quinoa to cool after cooking according to package instructions.
- In a bowl, combine cooked quinoa, black beans, diced bell peppers, cherry tomatoes, corn kernels, chopped cilantro, and a squeeze of lime juice.
- Drizzle with a simple dressing made from olive oil, lime juice, cumin, and salt.
- Toss everything together and let the flavors meld for a few minutes before enjoying the refreshing and satisfying salad mindfully.

Ratatouille:

- Sauté onions and garlic in a large pan with olive oil until translucent.

- Sliced eggplant, zucchini, bell peppers, and tomatoes should be added.
- Season with herbs like thyme, basil, and oregano, and let it simmer until the vegetables are tender.
- Serve the ratatouille as a standalone dish or with a side of crusty whole-grain bread or cooked quinoa.
- Appreciate the rich flavors and the medley of vegetables as you savor each bite.

Remember to customize these recipes based on your taste preferences and dietary needs. Embrace the process of cooking and preparing your dinner mindfully, and create a calming atmosphere to enjoy your meal. Savor the nourishment and the connection with your food as you eat slowly and with intention.

Mindful snack recipes

Enjoying mindful snacks throughout the day can provide a moment of nourishment and rejuvenation.

Here are some mindful snack recipes to inspire you:

Apple Slices with Nut Butter:

- Slice a fresh apple into thin rounds or wedges.
- Pair the apple slices with your choice of nut butter, such as almond butter or peanut butter.
- Sprinkle with a pinch of cinnamon or a drizzle of honey for added flavor.
- Savor each bite, appreciating the crispness of the apple and the creamy nut butter.

Trail Mix:

- Create a custom trail mix by combining a variety of nuts, seeds, and dried fruits.

- Choose your favorites, such as almonds, walnuts, pumpkin seeds, sunflower seeds, dried cranberries, and dried apricots.
- Mix them together in a bowl and portion out into small snack bags or containers.
- Enjoy the mix mindfully, noticing the different textures and flavors of each component.

Greek Yogurt Parfait:

- Layer Greek yogurt, fresh berries, and a sprinkle of granola or crushed nuts in a glass or bowl.
- Optional: Add a drizzle of honey or maple syrup for sweetness.
- Take your time to enjoy the creamy yogurt, the burst of fruity flavors, and the crunch of the granola.

Veggie Sticks with Hummus:

- Slice colorful vegetables like carrots, cucumber, bell peppers, and celery into sticks.

- Serve the veggie sticks with a side of hummus or another healthy dip of your choice.
- Enjoy the combination of crisp vegetables and creamy dip mindfully, appreciating the natural flavors and textures.

Energy Balls:

- In a food processor, combine dates, nuts (such as almonds, cashews, or walnuts), and a binder like almond butter or honey.
- Optional: Add other ingredients like cocoa powder, shredded coconut, or chia seeds for extra flavor and texture.
- Process until the mixture forms a sticky dough.
- Refrigerate until firm, then roll the mixture into bite-sized balls.
- When you have a snack craving, grab an energy ball and savor the sweetness and satisfying texture.

Remember, the purpose of mindful snacking is to cultivate awareness and appreciation for the food you eat. Choose snacks that are nourishing and satisfying, and take the time to enjoy each bite. Engage your senses, pay attention to the flavors and textures, and eat your snacks slowly and with intention.

Mindful dessert recipes

Ending your day with a mindful dessert can be a delightful way to unwind and treat yourself.

Here are some mindful dessert recipes to inspire you:

Dark Chocolate Dipped Strawberries:

- Melt dark chocolate (70% cocoa or higher) using a double boiler or microwave.
- Dip fresh strawberries into the melted chocolate, letting any excess drip off.
- Place the chocolate-dipped strawberries on a parchment-lined tray and refrigerate until the chocolate hardens.
- Enjoy each luscious bite mindfully, savoring the combination of juicy strawberry and rich dark chocolate.

Yogurt and Fruit Parfait:

- Layer Greek yogurt, sliced fresh fruits (such as berries, bananas, or mango), and a sprinkle of granola or crushed nuts in a glass or bowl.
- Optional: Drizzle with a small amount of honey or maple syrup for sweetness.
- Take your time to appreciate the colorful layers, the creamy yogurt, and the burst of fruity flavors.

Baked Apples with Cinnamon:

- Core and slice apples, leaving the skin intact.
- Place the apple slices in a baking dish and sprinkle with cinnamon and a touch of sweetener, like honey or maple syrup.
- Bake in the oven until the apples are tender and slightly caramelized.
- Serve the baked apples warm and enjoy the cozy flavors mindfully.

Chia Seed Pudding:

- In a jar or bowl, mix chia seeds with your choice of milk (such as almond milk, coconut milk, or dairy milk) and a sweetener like honey or agave syrup.
- Stir well and refrigerate overnight, or for at least a few hours until the chia seeds absorb the liquid and thicken.
- Top the chia seed pudding with fresh fruits, shredded coconut, or a sprinkle of nuts.
- Take your time to enjoy the creamy, pudding-like texture and the subtle sweetness of the chia seeds.

Banana Nice Cream:

- Peel and slice ripe bananas into chunks.
- Freeze the banana chunks until solid.
- Blend the frozen banana chunks in a food processor or blender until smooth and creamy, resembling ice cream.

- Optional: Add flavor variations like cocoa powder, vanilla extract, or a handful of frozen berries.
- Scoop the banana nice cream into a bowl or cone and enjoy the creamy and naturally sweet treat mindfully.

Remember to choose desserts that align with your mindful eating goals and preferences. Be present and fully engage your senses as you enjoy these treats. Eat your dessert slowly, savoring each bite and appreciating the indulgence in a mindful manner.

Chapter 4

Mindful Eating on the Go

Maintaining mindfulness while eating on the go can be a challenge, but with some preparation and intention, it's possible to cultivate mindful eating habits even in busy situations.

Here are some tips for practicing mindful eating on the go:

Plan Ahead:

- Take a few moments to plan your meals and snacks in advance.
- Pack nutritious and satisfying foods that are easy to eat on the go, such as pre-cut fruits and vegetables, nuts, seeds, or homemade energy bars.
- By having mindful food choices readily available, you can avoid relying on unhealthy convenience options.

Slow Down and Chew:

- When eating on the go, it's common to rush through meals. Slow down and take smaller bites.
- Chew your food thoroughly, savoring the flavors and textures. This aids digestion and allows you to truly enjoy your meal.

Mindful Snacking:

- Choose snacks that require more time to eat, such as nuts in their shells or a piece of fruit that needs peeling.
- By engaging in these small actions, you become more present and aware of the eating experience.

Create a Calm Environment:

- Find a peaceful spot, such as a park bench or a quiet corner, to sit and enjoy your meal.
- This allows you to focus on your food and surroundings rather than being distracted by external stimuli.

Disconnect from Distractions:

- Put away electronic devices and avoid multitasking while eating.
- By giving your full attention to your food, you can better tune into your body's hunger and fullness cues.

Appreciate the Senses:

- Engage your senses by noticing the colors, aromas, and flavors of your food.
- Take a moment to express gratitude for the nourishment and the effort that went into preparing the meal.

Practice Mindful Sips:

- If you're enjoying a beverage on the go, such as a cup of tea or a smoothie, take small sips and savor each one mindfully.
- Pay attention to the temperature, taste, and how it feels as it enters your body.

Listen to Your Body:

- Pay attention to your body's cues for hunger and fullness.
- Eat until you're satisfied, rather than overeating due to external cues or time constraints.

Remember, practicing mindful eating on the go is about finding balance and making conscious choices. Even in busy situations, take a moment to pause, connect with your food, and nourish your body and mind.

Tips for mindful eating when eating out

Eating out at restaurants can present challenges to mindful eating, as there are often distractions and tempting choices. However, with some mindful strategies, you can still make conscious choices and enjoy your dining experience.

Here are some tips for mindful eating when eating out:

Choose Your Restaurant Wisely:

- Look for restaurants that offer healthier options and prioritize fresh, whole ingredients.
- Seek out establishments that accommodate dietary preferences or restrictions, allowing you to make choices aligned with your goals.

Be Present and Mindful:

- Take a few moments to center yourself before ordering. Take deep breaths and set an intention to eat mindfully.
- Avoid distractions like phones or other electronic devices, and focus on the experience of dining.

Scan the Menu:

- Take time to read the menu thoroughly, paying attention to the ingredients and preparation methods.
- Look for dishes that include a balance of proteins, vegetables, and whole grains or starches.

Customize Your Order:

- Don't hesitate to request modifications to suit your preferences or dietary needs.
- Ask for dressings or sauces on the side, opt for steamed or grilled preparations, or substitute healthier sides.

Practice Portion Control:

- Be mindful of portion sizes, as restaurants often serve larger portions than necessary.
- Consider sharing a dish with a dining companion or ask for a take-out container to pack leftovers before you start eating.

Eat Slowly and Chew Thoroughly:

- Take your time to enjoy each bite, savoring the flavors and textures.
- Put your utensils down between bites, allowing yourself to fully chew and appreciate the food.

Engage Your Senses:

- Pay attention to the presentation of the food, its aroma, and how it appeals to your senses.
- Notice the colors, smells, and tastes, and appreciate the culinary experience.

Listen to Your Body:

- Pay attention to your body's cues for hunger and fullness.
- Eat until you're satisfied, rather than feeling obligated to finish everything on your plate.

Practice Mindful Socializing:

- Enjoy the company of your dining companions and engage in meaningful conversations.
- Avoid rushing through the meal and allow yourself to fully connect with the people you're dining with.

Practice Gratitude:

- Express gratitude for the food, the effort that went into preparing it, and the opportunity to dine out.

Remember, eating out should be an enjoyable experience. By approaching it with mindfulness, you can make conscious choices that align with your well-being while still savoring the pleasure of dining out.

Healthy and mindful fast food options

While fast food is often associated with unhealthy choices, there are increasingly more options available that can align with mindful and healthy eating habits.

Here are some healthier and mindful fast food options to consider:

Salad Bowls:

- Many fast food chains now offer customizable salad bowls with a variety of fresh vegetables, lean protein (such as grilled chicken or tofu), and nutritious toppings.
- Opt for lighter dressings on the side or choose vinegar-based dressings for a healthier option.

Grilled Options:

- Look for grilled chicken or fish sandwiches instead of fried options.

- Grilled items tend to be lower in fat and calories, making them a better choice for mindful eating.

Whole Grain Sandwiches or Wraps:

- Choose sandwiches or wraps made with whole grain bread or tortillas.
- Whole grains provide more fiber and nutrients compared to their refined counterparts.

Vegetable-Based Burgers:

- Several fast food chains now offer plant-based burgers made from vegetables or legumes.
- These options can be a healthier alternative to traditional beef burgers and still provide a satisfying meal.

Fresh Fruit Cups:

- Instead of opting for sugary desserts, look for fresh fruit cups or side options.

- These can provide natural sweetness and a dose of vitamins and minerals.

Yogurt Parfaits:

- Some fast food establishments offer yogurt parfaits with fresh fruit and granola.
- These can be a healthier choice for a satisfying and balanced snack or breakfast option.

Customizable Options:

- Look for fast food restaurants that allow you to customize your order.
- This way, you can control the ingredients and choose healthier options like extra vegetables, lean proteins, or whole grains.

Mindful Portion Control:

- Be mindful of portion sizes and avoid super-sized or combo meals.

- Opt for smaller-sized options or choose a regular-sized meal and pair it with a side salad or fresh fruit.

Remember, even when making healthier choices at fast food establishments, it's still important to be mindful of your overall dietary habits. Balance is key, and incorporating whole, unprocessed foods into your meals whenever possible is beneficial for your health.

Mindful travel snacks and meals

When traveling, having mindful snacks and meals on hand can help you stay nourished, energized, and make healthier choices.

Here are some ideas for mindful travel snacks and meals:

Fresh Fruit:

- Pack portable fruits like apples, oranges, bananas, or grapes that are easy to eat on the go.
- They provide natural sweetness, hydration, and essential vitamins and minerals.

Raw Vegetables and Dip:

- Cut up vegetables such as carrot sticks, celery, bell peppers, or cherry tomatoes.
- Pack them in a container with a small portion of hummus, guacamole, or Greek yogurt dip for added flavor and nutrients.

Trail Mix:

- Create your own trail mix by combining a mix of unsalted nuts (almonds, walnuts, cashews), seeds (pumpkin, sunflower), and dried fruits (raisins, cranberries, apricots).
- Be mindful of portion sizes as nuts and dried fruits can be high in calories.

Nut Butter and Whole Grain Crackers:

- Portion out individual servings of your favorite nut butter, such as almond or peanut butter, into small containers.
- Pair it with whole-grain crackers for a satisfying and balanced snack.

Protein Bars:

- Look for protein bars made with natural ingredients and minimal added sugars.
- Choose options that provide a good balance of protein, fiber, and healthy fats.

Yogurt Cups:

- Opt for single-serve containers of Greek yogurt or plant-based yogurt.
- Look for options with lower added sugars and consider packing a small bag of granola or nuts to sprinkle on top for added crunch.

Sandwiches or Wraps:

- Prepare homemade sandwiches or wraps using whole-grain bread or tortillas.
- Fill them with lean protein (such as grilled chicken, turkey, or tofu), vegetables, and a spread like hummus or avocado.

Pre-cut Vegetable Salad:

- Prepare a vegetable salad in advance with ingredients like mixed greens, cucumber, bell peppers, cherry tomatoes, and a light vinaigrette dressing.
- Pack it in a portable container to enjoy as a refreshing and nutritious meal on the go.

Hydration:

- Stay hydrated by carrying a refillable water bottle with you.
- Drinking enough water is essential for overall well-being and helps keep you alert and energized during your travels.

Remember, the key is to choose snacks and meals that are portable, nutritious, and satisfying. Be mindful of portion sizes, listen to your body's hunger and fullness cues, and aim for a balance of protein, fiber, and healthy fats to keep you fueled throughout your journey.

Chapter 5

Mindful Eating for Special Occasions

Special occasions often involve indulgent meals and treats, making it challenging to maintain mindful eating practices. However, with a mindful approach, you can still enjoy these occasions while staying connected to your body's needs.

Here are some tips for mindful eating during special occasions:

Set an Intention:

- Before the event, set an intention to approach the occasion with mindfulness.
- Remind yourself of your goals and values around health and well-being.

Engage Your Senses:

- Take a moment to appreciate the visual appeal, aromas, and flavors of the food.

- Slow down and savor each bite, fully experiencing the taste and textures.

Practice Portion Control:

- Mindfully choose smaller portions of indulgent foods, allowing yourself to enjoy the flavors without overindulging.
- Be aware of portion sizes and take note of your body's hunger and fullness cues.

Balance Your Plate:

- Aim to create a balanced plate by including a variety of vegetables, lean proteins, whole grains, and smaller portions of indulgent foods.
- Fill your plate with nutrient-dense options to help satisfy your hunger and nourish your body.

Mindful Indulgence:

- If there are particular treats or dishes you look forward to, allow yourself to enjoy them mindfully.
- Savor each bite and notice the sensations and satisfaction it brings.

Practice Mindful Socializing:

- Engage in meaningful conversations and connect with the people around you.
- Focus on the social aspect of the occasion rather than solely on the food.

Listen to Your Body:

- Pay attention to your body's signals of hunger and fullness throughout the event.
- Take breaks, drink water, and check in with yourself to determine if you're truly hungry or if you're satisfied.

Be Kind to Yourself:

- Remember that special occasions are meant to be enjoyed.
- If you find yourself overindulging, practice self-compassion and let go of any guilt or judgment.
- Instead, focus on making mindful choices moving forward.

Stay Active:

- Incorporate physical activity into your day, whether it's going for a walk, dancing, or engaging in a fun activity.
- Movement can help balance out indulgences and make you feel more energized.

Practice Gratitude:

- Take a moment to express gratitude for the food, the company, and the overall experience of the special occasion.
- Cultivating a sense of gratitude can help you appreciate and savor the moment.

Remember, special occasions are meant to be enjoyed, and practicing mindfulness during these times can help you make conscious choices and truly savor the experience. By being present and tuning into your body's cues, you can find a balance between indulgence and mindful eating.

Mindful eating during holidays and celebrations

Holidays and celebrations often involve an abundance of food and festivities, making it important to approach them with mindfulness and balance.

Here are some tips for practicing mindful eating during holidays and celebrations:

Set Intentions and Prioritize Balance:

- Before the holiday or celebration, set intentions to approach the occasion with mindfulness and balance.
- Remind yourself of your goals for overall well-being and maintaining a healthy relationship with food.

Be Selective and Mindful of Your Choices:

- Survey the food options available and choose mindfully.

- Opt for whole, unprocessed foods whenever possible and balance them with smaller portions of indulgent treats.

Practice Portion Control:

- Pay close attention to portion sizes and listen to your body's hunger and fullness cues.
- Serve yourself smaller portions and take your time to savor each bite.

Engage Your Senses:

- Take a moment to appreciate the colors, aromas, and textures of the food.
- Eat slowly and savor the flavors, allowing yourself to fully enjoy the experience.

Create a Balanced Plate:

- Aim to include a variety of vegetables, lean proteins, whole grains, and smaller portions of indulgent foods.

- Fill your plate with nutrient-dense options to help satisfy your hunger and nourish your body.

Practice Mindful Indulgence:

- Allow yourself to enjoy small portions of your favorite holiday treats or indulgent dishes.
- Savor each bite and fully experience the flavors and enjoyment they bring.

Mindful Socializing:

- Focus on the social aspect of the holiday or celebration, connecting with loved ones and engaging in meaningful conversations.
- Shift the focus from solely the food to the overall experience and connections.

Manage Stress:

- Holidays and celebrations can sometimes bring stress or emotional triggers.

- Be mindful of emotional eating and find healthy ways to manage stress, such as deep breathing, going for a walk, or practicing relaxation techniques.

Practice Self-Compassion:

- Be kind to yourself and let go of any guilt or judgment surrounding food choices.
- Remember that the occasional indulgence is a normal part of celebrations, and it's important to practice self-compassion and forgiveness.

Focus on Non-Food Activities:

- Plan and engage in non-food-related activities during the holiday or celebration.
- This can include playing games, going for a hike, or engaging in other enjoyable experiences that don't revolve around eating.

Remember, the goal of mindful eating during holidays and celebrations is to find a balance between enjoyment and nourishment. By practicing mindfulness, self-awareness, and moderation, you can fully experience the festivities while maintaining a healthy relationship with food.

Mindful eating at parties and social gatherings

Parties and social gatherings can present challenges for mindful eating, as they often involve a variety of tempting foods and a less structured eating environment. However, with some mindful strategies, you can still navigate these situations and make conscious choices.

Here are some tips for practicing mindful eating at parties and social gatherings:

Set an Intention:

- Before attending the event, set an intention to approach it with mindfulness and make conscious choices about what and how you eat.
- Remind yourself of your goals for well-being and nourishing your body.

Survey the Food Options:

- Take a moment to observe all the food options available before making your choices.
- Assess the options and select the ones that align with your health goals and preferences.

Start with a Balanced Plate:

- Fill your plate with a variety of foods, including vegetables, lean proteins, whole grains, and smaller portions of indulgent treats.
- Aim for a balanced combination of nutrients to satisfy your hunger and nourish your body.

Eat Mindfully:

- Slow down and savor each bite, paying attention to the flavors, textures, and sensations of the food.
- Chew slowly and fully before taking the next bite.

Be Mindful of Portion Sizes:

- Be aware of portion sizes and take smaller servings of indulgent foods.
- Enjoy them in moderation, allowing yourself to savor the taste without overindulging.

Listen to Your Body:

- Pay attention to your body's hunger and fullness cues throughout the event.
- Take breaks between bites, check in with yourself, and eat until you are comfortably satisfied, rather than overly full.

Practice Socializing:

- Engage in meaningful conversations and connect with the people around you.
- Concentrate on the social aspect of the gathering rather than solely on the food.

Stay Hydrated:

- Drink water throughout the event to stay hydrated and help maintain a sense of fullness.
- Choose water or unsweetened beverages rather than sugary drinks.

Limit Alcohol Consumption:

- Be mindful of alcohol consumption, as it can impair judgment and lead to overeating.
- Pace yourself, alternate with non-alcoholic beverages, and be aware of the potential impact on your mindful eating choices.

Practice Self-Compassion:

- If you find yourself not making the healthiest choices or overindulging, practice self-compassion.
- Remember that occasional indulgences are a normal part of social gatherings, and it's okay to enjoy them in moderation.

Remember, the goal is to find a balance between enjoying the social gathering and honoring your well-being through mindful eating. By being present, making conscious choices, and listening to your body's cues, you can navigate parties and social gatherings in a way that supports your health and enjoyment.

How to handle emotional eating triggers

Emotional eating refers to the practice of using food as a means to cope with or suppress emotions, rather than eating in response to physical hunger. It can be challenging to handle emotional eating triggers, but with mindfulness and alternative strategies, you can develop healthier coping mechanisms.

Here are some tips to help you manage emotional eating triggers:

Increase Self-Awareness:

- Take the time to recognize and understand your emotional eating triggers.
- Pay attention to the emotions, situations, or thoughts that tend to lead to emotional eating episodes.

Practice Mindfulness:

- Develop a mindful eating practice to cultivate awareness of your thoughts, feelings, and physical sensations related to eating.
- Pause before reaching for food and ask yourself if you are truly physically hungry or if it's an emotional craving.

Find Alternative Coping Strategies:

- Identify and experiment with alternative ways to manage your emotions without resorting to food.
- Engage in activities that bring you joy, such as practicing a hobby, reading, meditating, taking a walk, or journaling.

Build a Support Network:

- Seek support from friends, family, or professionals, such as therapists or support groups, to help you navigate emotional challenges.

- Having someone to talk to or lean on during difficult times can provide emotional support and help you manage triggers.

Practice Self-Care:

- Make self-care activities that nourish your mind, body, and soul a priority.
- Engage in activities like exercise, getting enough sleep, practicing relaxation techniques, or engaging in activities you enjoy.

Create a Food and Mood Diary:

- Keep a journal to track your eating patterns and emotions.
- Note down the triggers, emotions experienced, and food choices made during emotional eating episodes.
- This can help you identify patterns and gain insight into your emotional eating habits.

Distinguish Between Physical and Emotional Hunger:

- Learn to differentiate between physical and emotional hunger cues.
- Ask yourself if you are eating out of physiological hunger or as a response to emotional triggers.

Build a Balanced and Nourishing Diet:

- Focus on consuming a balanced diet with regular meals that include lean proteins, whole grains, fruits, vegetables, and healthy fats.
- Adequate nutrition can support overall emotional well-being and reduce the likelihood of emotional eating.

Practice Self-Compassion:

- Be kind to yourself and practice self-compassion.
- Accept that emotional eating is a common struggle and that it takes time and effort to develop healthier habits.

Seek Professional Help if Needed:

- If emotional eating persists and significantly affects your well-being, consider reaching out to a therapist or counselor who specializes in emotional eating or disordered eating patterns.
- They can provide guidance, support, and additional strategies tailored to your specific needs.

Remember, managing emotional eating triggers is a process that requires patience, self-compassion, and a commitment to developing healthier coping mechanisms. With practice and support, you can gradually shift your relationship with food and find healthier ways to address and manage your emotions.

Conclusion

In conclusion, mindful eating is a simple but powerful practice that can help you develop a healthier relationship with food. By being present and aware of your food choices, hunger and fullness cues, and the sensations in your body, you can make more informed decisions about what to eat, when to eat, and how much to eat. This book has provided you with a variety of tools, exercises, and recipes to help you get started on your mindful eating journey.

Remember that mindful eating is a process, not a destination and that every meal is an opportunity to practice and learn. By incorporating these practices into your daily life, you can enjoy a more nourishing, satisfying, and enjoyable relationship with food.

How to continue practicing mindful eating in your daily life

To continue practicing mindful eating in your daily life, here are some strategies and tips:

- **Set reminders**

Place visual cues or set alarms throughout the day to remind yourself to pause, check in with your body, and eat mindfully.

- **Create a peaceful eating environment**

Clear distractions and create a calm and inviting space for meals. Turn off screens, sit at a table, and create a pleasant atmosphere that encourages mindful eating.

- **Slow down**

Take your time to eat, savoring each bite. Chew slowly and thoroughly, allowing yourself to fully experience the flavors, textures, and sensations of the food.

- **Tune into your body**

Before eating, check in with your body to identify hunger and fullness cues. Eat when you are physically hungry and stop when you are comfortably satisfied.

- **Engage your senses**

Pay attention to the colors, aromas, and tastes of the food. Notice the textures and how each bite feels in your mouth. Engaging your senses enhances the mindful eating experience.

- **Practice portion control**

Be mindful of portion sizes and serve yourself appropriate amounts of food. Use smaller plates and bowls to visually trick your brain into feeling satisfied with less.

- **Practice gratitude**

Express gratitude for the food you are about to eat, the people involved in its preparation, and the nourishment it provides your body. Cultivating gratitude can enhance the mindful eating experience.

- **Mindful snacking**

Extend mindfulness to your snacking habits. Instead of mindlessly munching, take a moment to select a snack mindfully, savor it, and be fully present during the eating experience.

- **Reflect on your food choices**

Consider the nutritional value and the impact on your well-being when making food choices. Choose whole, unprocessed foods that nourish your body and support your health goals.

- **Practice self-compassion**

If you find yourself slipping into old habits or having an off day, practice self-compassion. Accept that mindful eating is a journey, and treat yourself with kindness and understanding.

- **Seek support and accountability**

Consider joining a mindful eating group, finding an accountability partner, or sharing your journey with friends and family. Having support can help you stay motivated and committed to your mindful eating practice.

Remember, practicing mindful eating is about cultivating awareness, presence, and a non-judgmental attitude towards your eating experiences. Every meal is an opportunity to reconnect with your body and make conscious choices that nourish you from the inside out. By integrating these mindful eating principles into your daily life, you can foster a healthier and more mindful relationship with food.

Final thoughts and words of encouragement

As you embark on your journey of mindful eating, remember that it is a personal and ongoing process. Be patient with yourself and embrace the opportunity to learn and grow along the way. It's normal to have moments of challenge or slip-ups, but every small step towards mindfulness is a step in the right direction.

Approach your relationship with food with curiosity, self-compassion, and a sense of adventure. Allow yourself to fully experience the joy of nourishing your body and savoring the flavors and textures of your meals. Embrace the mindfulness practices and techniques shared in this book, adapting them to suit your unique needs and preferences.

Remember that mindful eating goes beyond just the act of eating—it extends to how you approach food, how you engage with your senses, and how you cultivate a positive mindset around nourishment. It's about nurturing a deep connection with yourself and honoring your body's wisdom.

By practicing mindful eating, you have the opportunity to transform your relationship with food, enhance your overall well-being, and develop a greater sense of self-awareness. Embrace the journey, celebrate your progress, and enjoy the benefits that mindful eating can bring to your life.

Wishing you a fulfilling and nourishing mindful eating journey ahead!